Fitness for Men Over 40

Stay Fit and Healthy Through Middle Age

RON KNESS

Contents

Disclaimer

This publication is for informational purposes only and is not intended as medical advice. Medical advice should always be obtained from a qualified medical professional for any health conditions or symptoms associated with them.

Every possible effort has been made in preparing and researching this material. We make no warranties with respect to the accuracy, applicability of its contents or any omissions.

See your healthcare professional before starting any diet or exercise program!

Introduction

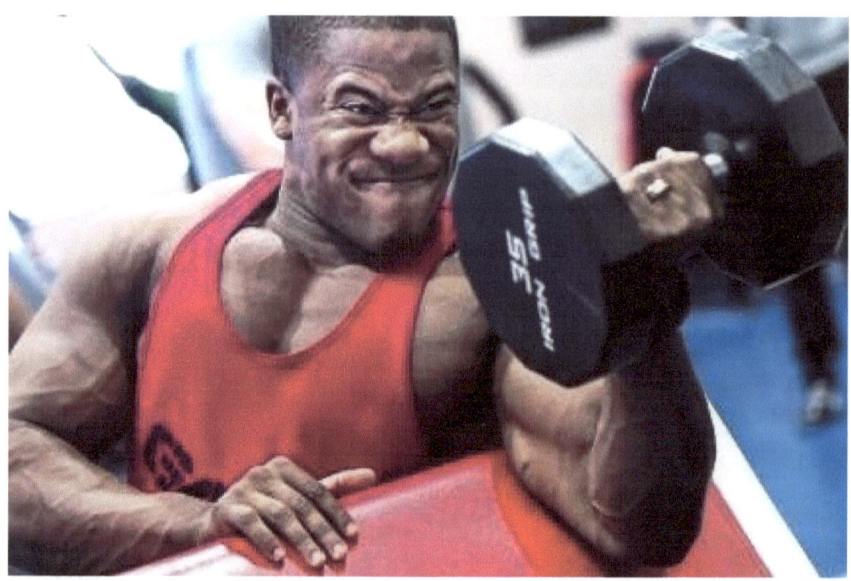

A question I frequently hear asked is *"Why do men over the age of 40 struggle to lose weight?"* And it is a fair question. That was about the time in my life when I had to start watching my weight. Now that I'm 65, it isn't getting any easier either as the years tick by. But with a lot of work, it is doable to keep your weight down and fitness level up. The chapters in this book show you how.

If you're a male in your forties or older, you definitely know the struggle is real. It doesn't matter if you were an athlete back in college or even a soldier back in the day as I was for 36 years … you will notice changes in your body.

You'll find it easier to gain weight and more difficult to lose it. If you do workout, you'll find it more difficult to do the same things you used to do with ease. The weights will seem heavier. Your stamina will have dropped. You'll feel less energetic and driven.

The only consolation here is that whatever you may be feeling is very normal. It's part and parcel of aging. Let's look at why a man has a tougher time losing weight once he crosses forty.

Drop in metabolism

This happens to everyone as they age regardless of gender. Your metabolic rate determines how fast your body burns calories. Young people, usually have a higher metabolic rate. Some people still manage to have a high metabolic rate even when they age and this is due to genetics.

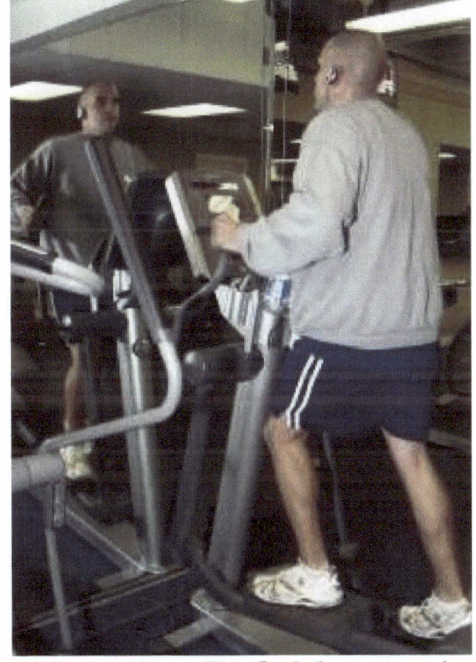

The only way to raise your metabolic rate will be to engage in high intensity training and eat foods that boost your metabolism naturally. Gaining muscle mass will help too, although it is difficult to gain let alone maintain.

Muscle atrophy

After the age of 35, most men will start to lose about 5% muscle mass every 10 years. This may not seem like much but it has an effect on the body. When you lose muscle mass, not only will you lose strength, but you'll also burn fewer calories while at rest. In part, responsible for weight gain.

Muscle is metabolically expensive. The more muscle you have, the higher your resting metabolic rate. This means you will be able to burn fat faster and also more easily.

Since men above 40 are losing muscle and burning fewer calories, this is a double whammy. They gain more fat and become weaker. The only way to counteract this problem will be to engage in resistance training to retard the muscle loss and try to reverse the process.

Sedentary lifestyle and stress

Most men usually focus more on their careers as they age. Exercise and fitness take a backseat as they strive to earn more and provide for their families. With this comes the stress of a hectic lifestyle and pressures from work.

Stress causes the body to release cortisol which indirectly leads to weight gain. Over and above that, since they're so busy and exhausted at work, most men just plop themselves on the couch, watch TV and eat unhealthy food once they're home.

This sedentary lifestyle causes them to gain weight over time. Before they know it, they're obese, have a huge belly to deal with and out of shape.

The only way to fix this problem will be to make your lifestyle more active. You'll need to dedicate thirty minutes to an hour per day specifically for exercise. You must make it a part of your daily routine, rather than an afterthought, if you have the time and energy left at the end of the day.

To do this, it's best to exercise first thing in the morning before you start your day or go to work. This way, you'd have gotten it out of the way and will not be too exhausted to exercise later. You'd also raise your body's metabolic rate and put it in fat burning mode for the rest of the day.

These are some of the most common reasons men gain weight after forty. There are other reasons but these are the big three. Most men would solve their weight gain issues just by eliminating these three causes. It can be done if you work on it.

4 Weight Loss Tips for Middle-aged Men

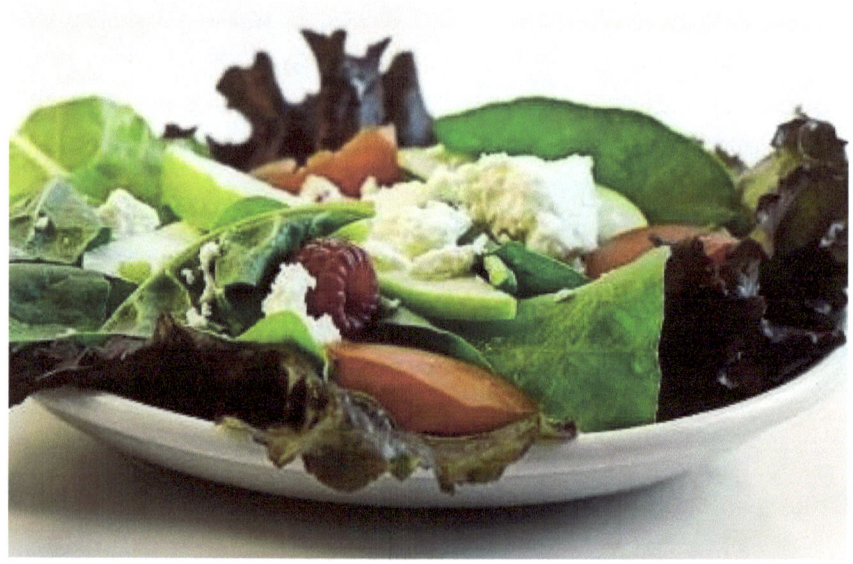

While the weight loss tips in this chapter can be applied to people of all ages and genders, it is tweaked to "middle-aged" men is because we face challenges that younger people don't. By using these tips, we'll be able to compensate for the effects of aging and lose weight more effectively.

Weight loss is a journey, not necessarily a destination – there is no ending point. And you're not going to get there overnight. Depending on how overweight you are, it can take you anywhere from 30 to 90 days to see amazing results. Some seriously obese people may take up to 6 months or even a year to reach their ideal weight.

What matters here is not the time that it takes. The time is going to pass anyway.

What matters is that you stay the course. Even if the results come at a snail's pace, as long as you stay on track, keep moving, making progress and apply the tips below, you will succeed.

Reduce your carbs

This is the most powerful tip of the lot. As you age, your metabolism drops and you burn fewer calories throughout the day. Carbs are calorie dense and it's extremely difficult to burn off these calories if you're not active enough. It stands to reason that is you eat the same amount of food, but are not burning off the same number of calories, you are going to gain weight.

Furthermore, carbs start off a chain of processes in the body that involve raising your blood sugar levels and causing insulin insensitivity. This translates to fat bcing shuttled off to be stored for future use.

It's best to reduce your consumption of bread, pasta, white rice, etc. Veggies are a source of good carbs and you can consume them freely. Just avoid the man-made carbs.

Do resistance training

You absolutely must build muscle in order to raise your metabolic rate. The more muscle you have, the more 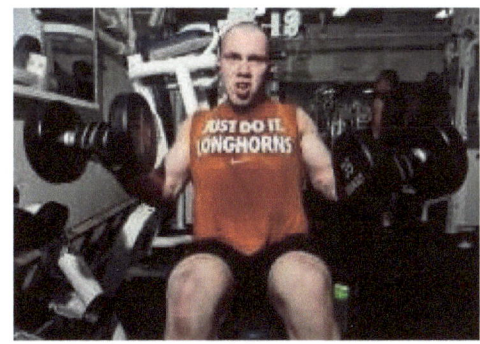 calories you will burn, even while at rest and sleeping.

It is actually ironic that most males are interested in building muscles and looking good when they're young but once they're married, they let themselves go.

When you're young, you do not lose muscle easily. However, after the age of 35, you lose muscle every year – as mentioned earlier at the rate of 5% every 10 years. So... it is MUCH MORE IMPORTANT to at least keep the muscle mass you currently have and even try to gain muscle when you're in your forties and above.

By building your muscles, your resting metabolic rate will increase and you'll be less likely to gain weight and more likely to lose fat.

Do intermittent fasting

This is a very powerful method of losing weight. Basically, all you will be doing is consuming your daily caloric intake within a fixed time frame. If your eating window is 6 hours long, you'll consume all your calories during these 6 hours. After that you will not eat till the next day.

You won't be starving yourself because you're getting your daily calories. However, your body will have a much longer time to be in a fasted state and use calories from its fat stores instead of burning food for fuel. You will lose more fat in this way.

High intensity training

It would be a great idea to get programs such as P90X by Tony Horton or Insanity Max by Shaun T. These are NOT easy programs but there are modifier moves for those who are not as fit to follow.

The intensity of these programs will boost your metabolic rate and create a situation in your body known as excess post-exercise oxygen consumption. So, even though the workout may only last 30 minutes, your body will be in fat burning mode for 6 to 12 hours after that.

You will be a fat burning machine round the clock. Of course, approach the training sensibly and cautiously. Exert till you're exhausted but don't push yourself so hard that you end up fainting.

Pressure may turn coal into diamonds... but it also turns it to dust. Exercise smart!

The key to losing weight is to make incremental and measurable progress with time. If you stick to the program for 90 days, there is absolutely no doubt that you will lose weight. You're never too old to start... so get started today.

7 Workout Tips for Men Over 40

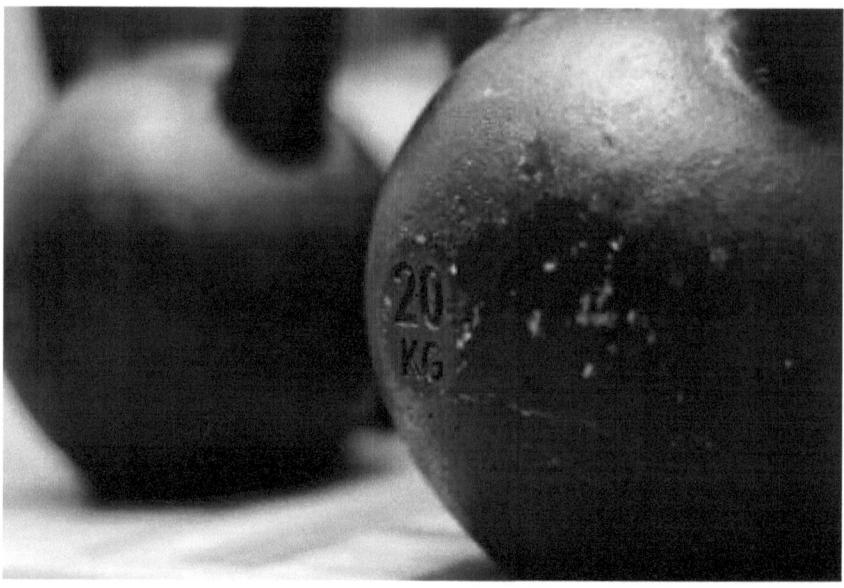

Training methods don't really change much despite your age. In fact, they don't really differ between sexes either.

If you want to retain and build muscle, you need to engage in resistance training a couple days per week …just make sure they are not consecutive days. To improve your stamina and endurance, you need cardio sessions four times a week. On the seventh day rest, so your body has time to repair itself. To lose weight, you need to be at a caloric deficit – consuming around 500 fewer calories per day than you burn.

These are the basic principles that apply whether you're 18 or 80. However, as one ages, the joints become less mobile and the muscles lose some flexibility. This is inevitable.

The only way to retard this aging process will be to start exercising while young and carry on being active right up into your golden years.

There is a reason why action stars like Sylvester Stallone and Dwayne Johnson (the Rock) still look so fit and tough while many men their age look flabby or like withered prunes.

It's the constant exercise. They never let themselves go. To be active in your later years, you need to stay active all the way.

If you're just getting started, cast your worries aside. It is never too late to improve. You'll be amazed at how much progress you can make with consistency and determination.

This chapter gives you 7 tips that men above 40 should be aware of. While the principles may not change, your body does and you must know how to compensate for any loss of flexibility or other limitations.

Cardio

If you're trying to lose weight, you absolutely need cardio.
Cardio will boost your metabolic rate, increase your stamina and have a whole host of other health and fitness benefits. As you age, very often you'll find you get winded more easily.

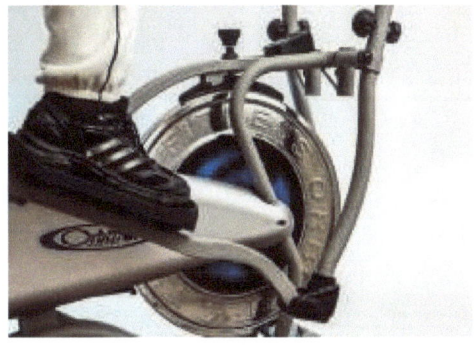

Do NOT push yourself to the point where you're throwing up. The old adages of "Go hard or go home" and "No pain, no gain" do not apply here.

Take your time to make gradual improvements. It would be a good idea to get programs like P90X or Insanity to help you or do a HIIT routine. These programs are structured and you can follow along.

You do not need to keep up if you're gasping and totally exhausted. You just need to do your best, rest a bit and carry on.

Heavier weights

Generally, men who are 40 and above, have lots of responsibilities, such as their careers and families. You want your workouts to be short and effective.

Since you want to preserve or even try to increase muscle mass, the best way to go about this is to use the maximum amount of weight that you can move with good form. Aim for 6 to 8 reps. There is no need to do countless reps. That builds endurance, but not mass. Just aim for 4 to 5 sets of 6 to 8 reps per set.

Give yourself adequate time to recover; never do the same strength training routines two days back-to-back. Give yourself at least a day in between, unless you are working a totally different set of muscles.

Focus on compound movements instead of isolation exercises. Compound movements bring more muscles into play. Pull-ups will always be better than preacher curls for you. If you have the time, then sure… go ahead and do the isolation exercises.

If not, stick to the exercises that work several muscle groups at once and use as much weight as you can safely can manage.

Stretch and warm up well

Always stretch sufficiently before and after a workout. Before you do any resistance training, always engage in some light cardio for about 5 minutes just to warm up the muscles.

Jumping jacks, light running on the treadmill, light skipping a jump rope, etc. are good ways to warm up your muscles.

Note there is a difference between stretching and warming up. Do not stretch too much before a resistance training workout or your performance will suffer.

As far as stretching, do dynamic stretching before working out and static stretching after a workout. Dynamic stretching works a muscle through its range of motion, whereas static stretching holds the muscle in the stretched position.

Longer rest periods

Rest sufficiently between sets and between workouts. If your muscles are in pain, give them a rest and wait till they heal. It takes longer as you age. So, be patient and gentle with your body.

More controlled and less explosive

Keep your resistance training more controlled and less explosive. Many men experience injuries, such as strains and sprains because their movements are jerky and their bodies are not conditioned enough to handle the explosive movements. If you are new to strength training, weight machines may be a better option to start with until you get the feel for using weights. It is easier with free weights to lose control and either hurt yourself or someone around you.

Don't try to do deadlifts fast and throw out your back. Have good form and train safely.

Diet

Since there will be some limitations as you age, your training will be affected. This is something you can't control. What you can control however, is your diet. Eat clean and exercise good portion control.

If your diet is on point, you will look healthy and feel healthy. If your diet is haphazard, you will gain weight, have less energy and be opening yourself up to possible health issues. We cover some on diet in the next chapter.

Attitude

You know what they say… "Your attitude determines your altitude." This is very true. You must be positive and believe that you can do it.

Do not assume that you're old just because you're above forty. You can always reclaim your health and body if you put in the effort. You'll be amazed at what you can achieve with consistency and time.

Many top bodybuilders peak in their forties. The actors in The Expendables are mostly above 40. They're still fit and strong.

Keep your chin up, dig your heels in the dirt and tell yourself that you can be fit. It can be done… and you will start today.

The Best Diet for Men to Build Muscle

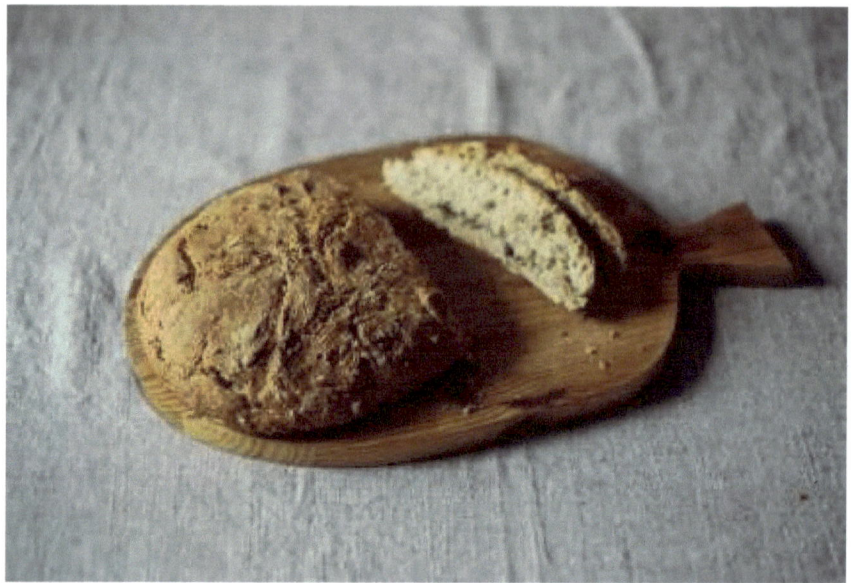

When it comes to nutritional needs, the best diet for men to build muscle includes a balance of complex carbohydrates and proteins. It might surprise you to know that the diet for men to build muscle is really not all that different from the diet for women.

Where you'll see the biggest difference for the sexes is in the calorie requirements. Men can require up to a thousand or more calories each day than women do in order to build muscle mass. But other than that, men don't really have any special requirements based on their gender.

Here are some important factors to consider when choosing the best diet for your muscle training program.

Whole Foods. The best sources of nutrients come from whole foods. You'll want to fill your diet with whole grains, lean meats, nuts, eggs, fruits, and vegetables in order to build muscle efficiently.

Increase Your Calories. When you begin a strenuous workout program, you'll be using more energy. If you don't add more calories to your diet, your body may not have enough energy to build muscle during the recovery phase.

When you're trying to build muscle, it isn't the right time to restrict calories. However, if you notice that you're adding fat to your body you may need to lower your caloric intake.

Pay attention to your body's signals as you look for the right calorie/workout balance.

Add Protein. While you can get a lot of protein from both animal and plant sources in the food you cat, it's almost always helpful to add a protein supplement when you're weight training. You'll be asking a lot of your body to repair and rebuild tissues and you'll need extra protein.

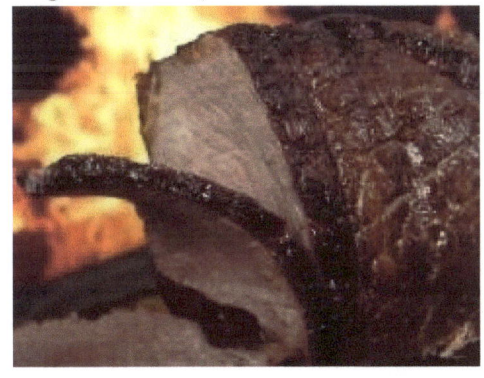

You can look for a protein powder made from whey, soy, egg, or even rice. Whey protein is the easiest for your body to digest but if you're vegan or allergic to whey you may need to seek an alternative.

Eat All Day. As important as how much you eat is how often you eat. You need to eat several meals a day to keep your body from running out of fuel. This helps your metabolism stay strong and fast, and helps you to burn fat.

Allow a Few Treats. It's important to eat healthy, but you also have to allow yourself to enjoy some of your favorite foods. Try eating clean at least six days a week and allowing yourself one day each week to indulge (albeit small) in some other foods. This will keep you from quitting a healthy diet program.

The best diet for men to build muscle includes a balance of carbohydrates, proteins, and healthy fats at about a 50%,30%, 20%, respectively and is also packed with calories.

If You Are a Male, You Need to Read This!

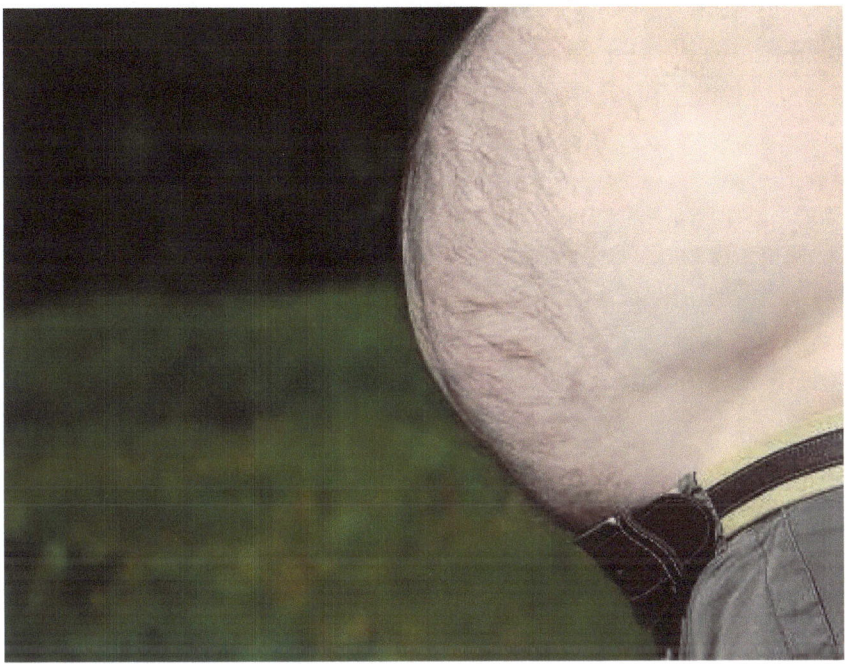

We live in an age where problems like diabetes, obesity and a plethora of other medical issues are at epidemic levels. Most of these problems are the result of poor dietary choices, a sedentary lifestyle and too much stress.

The good news is that all of these can be avoided if one takes the bull by the horns and actually takes action to put an end to the problem. However, in the times that we live in, excuses are made and an unhealthy lifestyle is actually glamorized.

The "Dad Bod" was all the rage some time back and the media and a few other clueless people were saying that such a body is attractive and it shows that a man is confident in his own skin and still healthy.

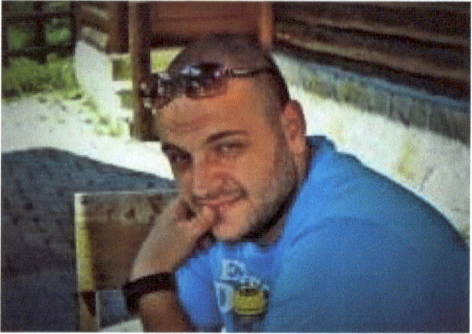

Nothing could be further from the truth. There is nothing healthy about a Dad Bod. Let's not worry about appearances for a minute. It's not about whether you have six pack abs or a plump appearance. Looks are not the issue here.

The repercussions on your health are. Most men with abdominal fat are exposing themselves to many possible health risks. The belly is one of the first places where men gain weight.

This explains why you often see many middle-aged men with huge bellies.

You must be aware there are two kinds of fat in the body. There is subcutaneous fat which is fat under the skin and there is visceral fat, which is fat that builds up in the spaces around your organs, such as the intestines and stomach.

It's this visceral fat that causes your body to store toxins and also causes inflammation. The dangerous part here is that even with a body that doesn't seem morbidly obese, you might have quite a lot of visceral fat stored in your organs.

This sets the stage for problems like diabetes, heart disease, inflammation and all the other problems that are just waiting for the right opportunity to strike. This is exactly why you need to be on guard at the gate. Just laughing off an out of shape body and calling it a cool trend will do you no favor once these diseases take root.

Always bear in mind – prevention is better than cure.

High blood sugar levels, high cholesterol levels, unexplained aches and pains all over the body, lethargy, depression and many other problems are the result of a poor diet and an inactive lifestyle.

You can keep many health problems at bay just by watching your diet, making the right food choices and getting daily exercise. Avoid the processed food, consume alcohol only on special occasions and take an active interest in your health.

Aging is a slow process and most men forget that with time, their bodies just can't cope with the ravages of an unhealthy lifestyle. The late night parties, instant noodles and lying on the couch playing video games for hours were fine when you were young ... well not really, but you did it anyway without thinking about the consequences later on in life.

However, as you age, the late nights at work, the tasty but unhealthy meals you consume and the hours spent watching TV (usually while eating unhealthy food) will not be as easily handled by your body. You're not old but you aren't that young anymore either.

This is a hard truth to come to terms with, but the sooner you do, the better. The foundation of all happiness is good health. Eat clean. Be active and live well.

Muscle Building Tips for Men Above 40

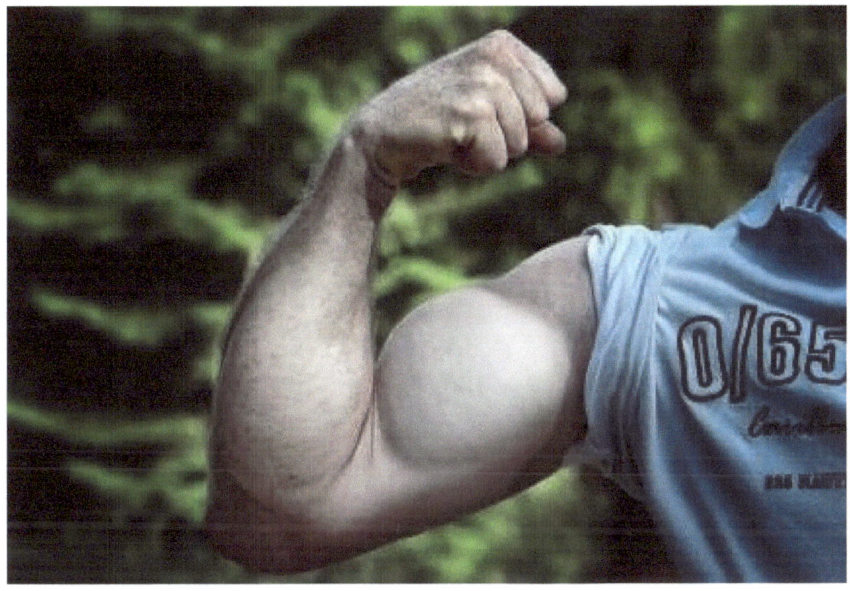

Contrary to popular belief, you can build muscle as you age. In fact, there are documented studies and photos of seniors in their fifties and even sixties who went on a weight training program and built muscle.

The photos showed amazing results and people half their ages aren't as ripped or muscular. So, it's never too late to take active steps to build muscle and look fit. It is just more hard to do after the age of 40.

Forty is not that old but there are a few differences that you must be aware of. First, it will take you longer to recover from your workouts. While you may have been able to train daily in your younger days, as you get older, your muscles take longer to recover.

Your upper body workout may leave you sore for 3 or 4 days. Recovery time will get better the longer you stick to a training program. But generally, just know that you don't have the 'healing powers' that you did in your twenties.

The way to work around this is to incorporate several different exercises during one workout. For example, you may work your chest, triceps, back and biceps on one day. On another day, you may work your legs, shoulders and forearms, etc.

This is just a rough idea. The point is you don't need to dedicate an entire day to training just one or two body parts. This can mean that you only need to use the gym three times a week instead of 5 to 6 times a week – at least in the beginning until you get used to working out. Remember the goal is to burn calories and you can't do that very well sitting on your butt watching TV.

Another point to note is that your joints may be more 'creaky' and less lubricated as they were when you were younger. So, it's best not to aim for countless reps. You want to move as much weight as possible, but by using good form. As noted before, you should aim for 3 sets in a 6 to 8 rep range per set.

There is no need to do hundreds of reps with light weights just to develop tone. It doesn't work that way. If your body fat percentage is low, there will be vascularity and your muscles will be defined.

The goal here is to do as much work as possible. Work done is equal to force multiplied by distance moved. In other words, in strength training terms simply move as much weight as you can.

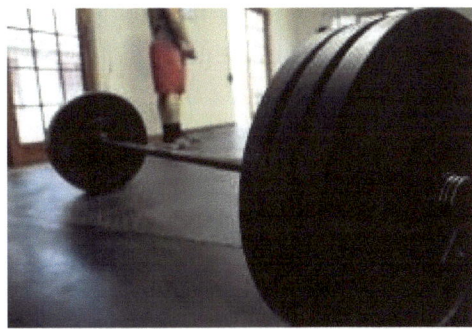

Always have rest periods in-between sets that are sufficient for you; generally around 90 seconds to two minutes between sets is enough. You do not need to do sets back to back without rest. Giving yourself time to catch your breath will allow you to execute better lifts with better form.

It would be a good idea to avoid explosive movements, such as superman push-ups, clean and jerk, etc. If you're new to training, your body will not be used to such moves and you may injure yourself. It's best to train gradually until you feel like you're capable of the more demanding exercises.

Many men, in an attempt at looking macho, take on more than they can handle. They end up throwing their backs out, straining a muscle or pulling a ligament… or do worse damage. Do things slow and steady.

This is an important point to remember. You must make incremental progress gradually over time. Check your ego at the door and train sensibly. Unless you have been training for years without falling into a sedentary lifestyle, it's best that you not be competitive with the younger folk at your gym.

Increase the weights gradually. Have good form. Train at least two times per week in the beginning, giving yourself sufficient time to recover.

If certain parts of your body ache, do exercises that don't tax those parts as heallvily.

As long as you understand your body and know that you are training for the long haul, you will see marvelous results in time. Stay the course and you will get there.

Five Ways to Build Muscle Mass After 40

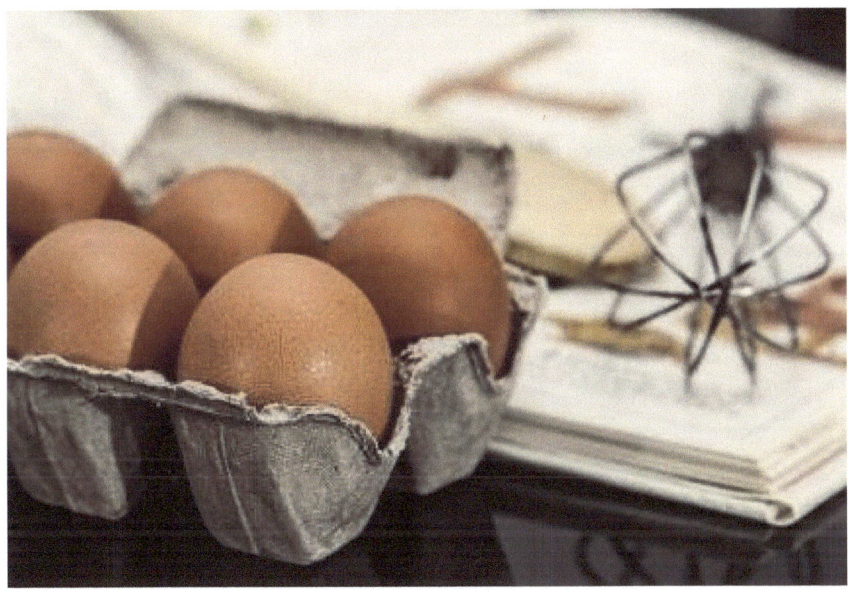

It gets more and more difficult to build muscle mass after 40. As you age, your body will naturally have a reduction in hormones that makes it harder to put on muscle mass and gain weight. But you can make lifestyle changes to build muscle regardless of your age.

Ramp up your protein. Often people over the age of 40 don't consume enough protein to truly support the building of muscle tissue. It's important to make sure that you're getting a serving of protein at each meal.

You can get protein from whole grains, meats, fish, beans, and nuts.

Dairy products such as milk, yogurt, and cheese can also provide you with plenty of protein. And if you still don't get enough, adding a protein shake or other type of protein supplement can be very beneficial.

Eat more food. You may have spent much of your life trying to eat fewer calories to maintain a healthy weight. But if you want to build muscle mass you'll have to reverse 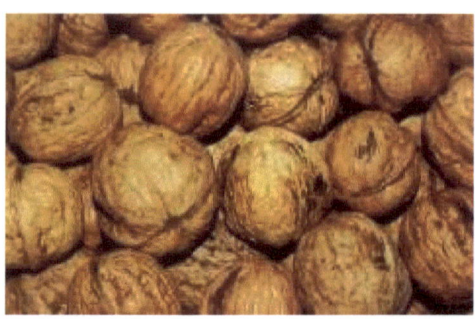 your thinking on this. It's important to provide your body with sufficient calories to build more mass.

That doesn't mean pigging out on your favorite junk foods. You still need to make sure that you get your extra calories from as many whole foods as possible. All calories are not created equal – you want to focus on good nutrition.

Cut back on alcohol. As you age, the effect alcohol can have increases. Drinking alcohol and using some types of drugs can cause your testosterone levels to plummet. You need a fairly high testosterone level in order to build muscle mass after age 40.

Make sure that you don't have any more than one or two drinks each day in order to protect your testosterone levels.

Participate in weight training. In order to build muscle, you have to use the ones you have. That means adding resistance training to your schedule at least twice a week. You should begin with exercises that use more than one muscle group such as squats, rowing, and bench press.

These will help you to exercise more parts of your body and allow you to spend less time at the gym while you increase your muscle mass quickly. It's important to make sure you follow proper form to protect your joints.

Get more rest. Your body builds muscle mass when you're resting. Especially when you're over 40, you need the rest to allow your body to produce the necessary hormone to grow your muscle tissue. But at an older age, you may get less sleep. Aim for 8-10 hours of sleep each night.

In order to build muscle mass after 40 you'll need to focus on making some lifestyle changes, but it is possible to have the best body of your life at this age.

The Best Exercise for Men In Their 40s and Above

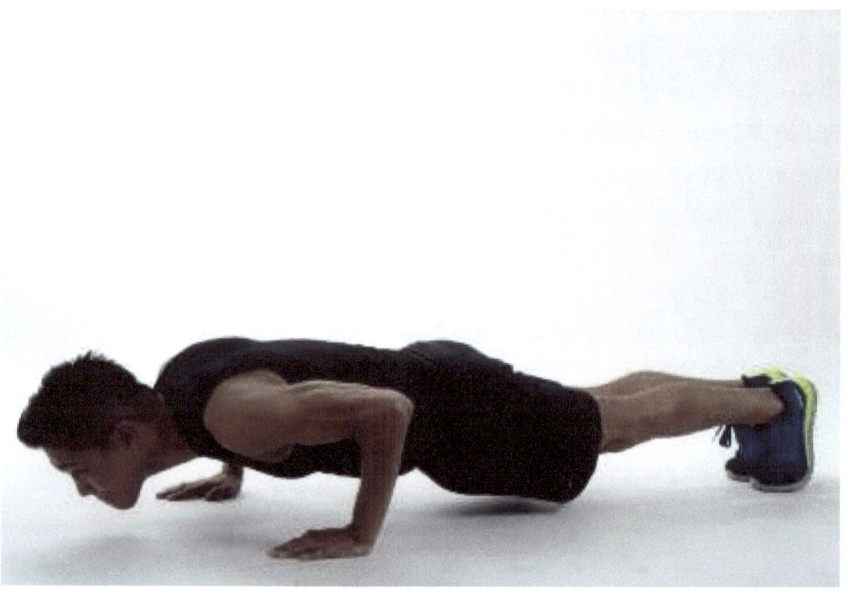

Men in their forties will see the best results if they focus on doing workouts that comprise of exercises which work several different muscle groups at once. This will not only be time efficient, but you'll be getting a full-body workout that will boost your metabolic rate and accelerate fat loss.

In fact, by lining up about 7 or 8 different exercises and doing them one after another with minimal rest, the entire workout will not only be a resistance training session but also a cardio session.

The majority of older men generally do not have hours to spend at the gym like younger guys who're trying to sculpt their bodies to turn girls' head.

Men in their forties have careers to get to, family responsibilities and a hundred and one other things to do.

They go to the gym to stay fit, build some muscle and look relatively good. The focus is less on the aesthetics and more on health. Since you want to be fit and strong with the least amount of time spent at the gym or in training, you really need to train hard and smart.

This chapter will give you some of the best exercises you should focus on. By mastering these moves, you will tone many muscle groups and add lean muscle faster. I've provided a YouTube video on how to do each exercise.

Pull-ups

https://youtu.be/swkOeoEcKW0

This is without a doubt, the benchmark of upper body strength. You'll be working your biceps, triceps, core, shoulders and back. Many men struggle to do just 10 pull-ups. Aim for 10 and then 15 and then 20.

This is achievable. Pull-ups are much more difficult to do than lat pulldowns which do not require as much core muscle engagement.

If you can't do any pull-ups, you can start by using a chair. Then you will do half pull-ups but lower yourself all the way down. After some time you will build enough strength to do many pull-ups without breaking a sweat.

Deadlift

https://youtu.be/RyJbvWAh6ec

Another fantastic must-do exercise. This exercise will work your back, legs, core and to a certain degree, your shoulders and arms. This is a very powerful exercise. Always do it with good form and lift as much weight as you possibly can safely. Aim for 8 reps and 3 to 4 sets.

Squat

https://youtu.be/nEQQle9-0NA

The benchmark of lower body strength. The squat will work your quads, core, calves and back. The more you work your leg muscles, the more calories you'll burn. Training the lower body is far more effective at accelerating fat loss.

Lunge burpees

https://youtu.be/5rHcNyWcNPc

These work your core, arms, legs and back. This exercise is often done by soldiers because of the full-body motion and it can be done fast to make it take on a cardio-like nature.

Push-ups

https://youtu.be/Eh00_rniF8E

Another great upper body exercise that works your core, triceps and chest. Do as many as you can till you reach failure.

Kettlebell snatches

https://youtu.be/-8JbTKR50rk

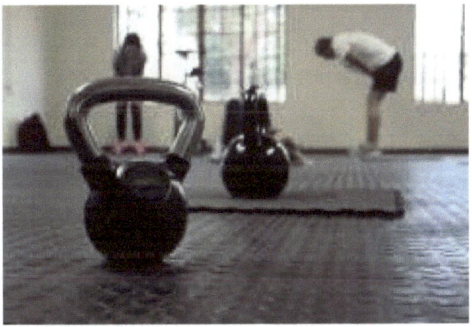

This move helps to strengthen many smaller muscles in the upper body. The stabilizing muscles in the body need a workout too and the kettlebell snatch does the job. Use controlled movements. This should not be done in an explosive manner.

Hanging leg raises

https://youtu.be/AEtTmtcBSOM

One of the best ab exercises. It also works the forearms and strengthens your grip. There is almost no impact with this exercise. Just make sure to control the leg raises and not jerk them up and down wildly. If leg raises seem too difficult, you can do knee raises.

Planks

https://youtu.be/TWpbe9nRySc

Forearm planks, side planks, straight planks, plank jacks, side plank crunches, etc. are some of the many ways you can tone your core and abs.

Learn as many different types of planks and do them in your workouts. You can find samples of each by searching YouTube.

They'll strengthen your core and your entire body will become stronger.

These are just some of the exercises that you can do. There are so many more out there. You may Google them or go on YouTube and look for more videos on how to do these exercises. As long as they're compound movements, not too jerky and dangerous, they will do just fine.

If you have any health issues or injuries, do speak to your doctor first before doing any exercise. Also, do err on the side of caution and stick to weights or moves that you can manage. Don't take on more than you can handle or you will end up hurting yourself.

Slow and steady wins the race. Use the exercises above to tone your body, look great and feel better than great.

Supplements for Men Over 40

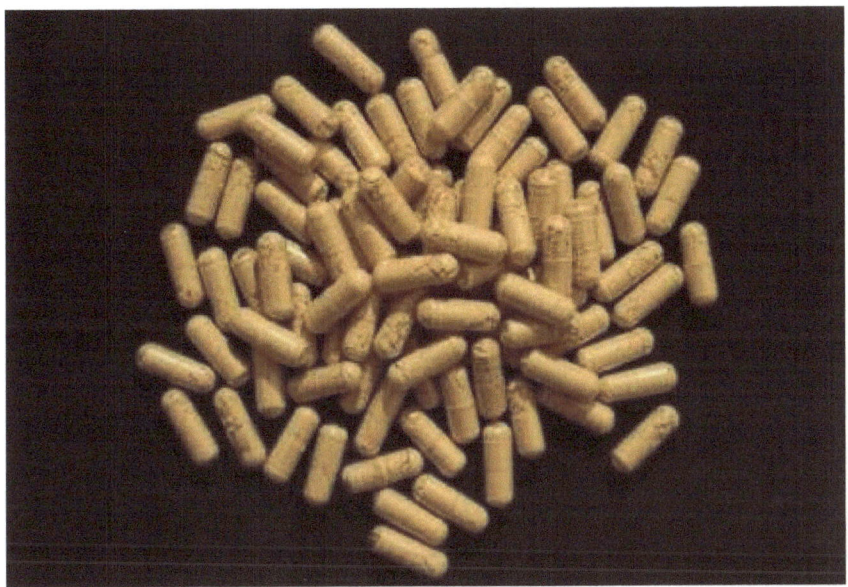

There is often much debate in the fitness industry about supplements. Are they safe? Should one take them? Do they work? Is it even necessary to waste your hard earned money on supplements?

In this chapter, we'll not just look at supplements that you can buy from stores that are rich in vitamins and nutrients which are beneficial to your body, but also ones you should get from natural food.

However, in some cases, you might need to consume a lot of a particular food just to get some specific nutrient. In cases like these, supplements in capsule or tablet are a great way to save time and effort. Just pop one pill or make a quick shake and you're good to go.

In this chapter we'll look at several different types of supplements that you should consider taking. Some are for your health, some are for recovery from exercise and some are to help you build muscle or lose fat.

Protein shakes

The most popular of all supplements, protein shakes have been around for ages. It can be egg protein, whey protein, soy protein, pea protein, etc. The main purpose of protein shakes is to give your body the protein it needs to build muscle and carry out other maintenance processes.

If you eat sufficient quantities of meat, broccoli, peas, lentils and other foods rich in protein, you may not need to consume protein shakes. The point is to get enough protein in whichever way you get it.

Protein is protein and natural sources are best. However, if you do not have time to watch your diet and see if you're getting sufficient protein, shakes are a quick and easy way to get your protein.

Creatine

Bodybuilders and guys trying to get buff swear by creatine and say then it makes their muscles bigger and look more "swole"… which is a term they use to describe nice, rounded muscles. While creatine is found in fish and meat, for you to see gains in strength and size, a creatine supplement will definitely help.

This is one of those supplements that actually work. If you're trying to build muscle and get a sculpted look (which is achievable even if you're 40 and above), you will definitely benefit with creatine.

Garlic pills

The allicin found in garlic is very potent and has medicinal properties that combat many health issues. It helps to reduce blood pressure, prevents common colds, reduces bad cholesterol levels, increases longevity, prevents Alzheimer's, etc.

It also helps improve athletic performance because it aids in recovery.

Instead of going through the torture of consuming tons of garlic, you can just swallow a garlic capsule daily and get your dose of this powerful antioxidant.

Fish oil

Our diets these days are too rich in Omega-6 fatty acids and don't contain enough Omega-3 fatty acids. This has led to most people having an imbalance of essential fatty acids. This is a huge problem and causes health issues like

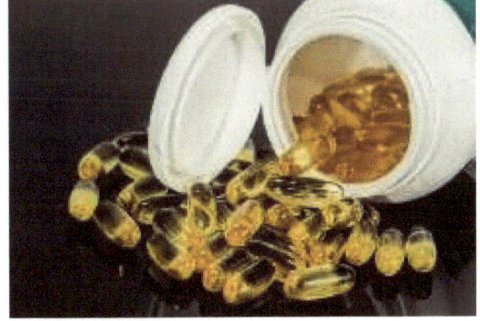

inflammation and other serious problems.

Most supplement stores will carry a variety of fish oil supplements such as cod liver oil capsules or krill oil supplements. Choose one that suits you best.

Nitric oxide

Nitric oxide helps with vasodilatation, which is just a big word that means it helps to expand your blood vessels. What this does is that it allows your muscles to get more oxygenated blood.

This will boost your performance during training and make you stronger. Your stamina will also improve by leaps and bounds. Just note that you need to take the supplements 30 minutes prior to your workout.

Greens food supplements

Despite Popeye's best efforts, the hard truth is that many adults hate their veggies too. Since veggies are chockfull of antioxidants and nutrients, you can't neglect your veggies.

One of the best ways to get them besides eating veggies will be to consume a greens food supplement, These greens powders or capsules usually contain nutrients from veggies such as wheat grass, barley, grains, vegetables, legumes, seaweed, nuts, herbs and much more.

You'll definitely benefit from consuming this supplement if you don't get enough veggies in your diet.

These are just some of the supplements that are great for your body. You don't need to go overboard and fret over all the different types of supplements out there. There are so many brands that it can be mind boggling.

Look for customer reviews before deciding on any one brand. Expensive doesn't necessarily mean it's the best. A lot of supplements are way overpriced because of the heavy advertising used by the manufacturers.

As long as the supplement has the right ingredients in the right quantity, it should do fine.

Test them out and always make sure that you eat a clean diet and lots of wholesome single ingredient foods. There is no supplement that can replace real food.

"Let food be thy medicine and medicine be thy food" - Hippocrates

Final Thoughts

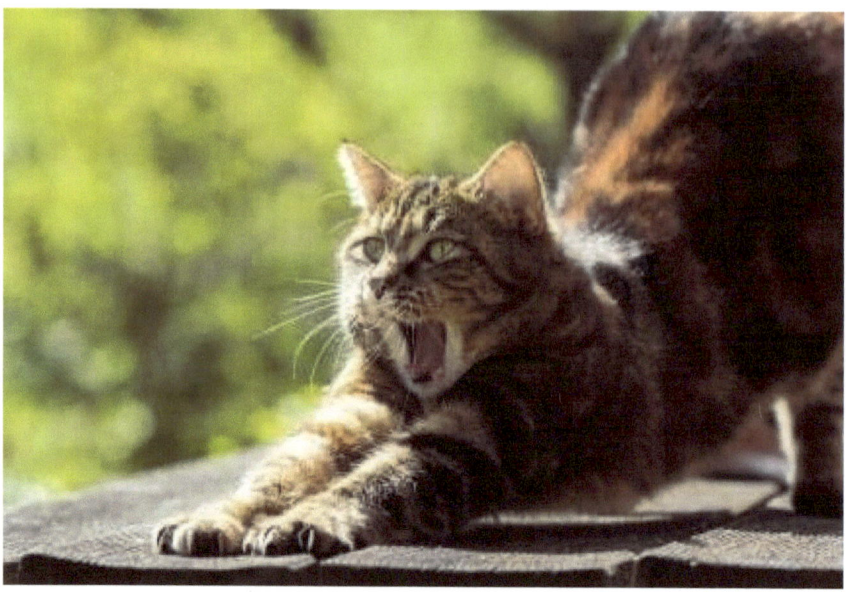

There are guidelines which you should keep in mind to remain injury free and active for years to come.

Be Conscious of Your Recovery Ability

It's old news, the older you are, the slower your recovery becomes. So, do not attempt to perform intense exercise 5 days a week. Instead, aim for a more balanced 2 days per week of resistance training; working the entire both on-days with sufficient rest between them (such as on Monday and then Thursday). By doing this, you allow your body enough time to recover from the previous session's workout.

In addition, perform low to moderate intensity cardiovascular exercise, using low impact methods. Best options including swimming, elliptical training, or cycling.

Set Realistic and Attainable Goals

If you're over 50, you will not gain pounds of lean mass every month, nor will you lose weight extremely fast. In fact, your body probably favors fat storage, and your metabolism is likely in pre-retirement. So, don't be disappointed if you do not make progress as fast as you'd expect, especially if you're new to training.

Your testosterone levels are weaning, as is growth hormone. Insulin sensitivity is likely poorer, and you may have concomitant diseases. Try to focus on consistency first, then let intensity follow.

Stretches Are Now Mandatory

No longer can you get away with lackluster or no stretches at all, at this point in time, stretches are necessary to keep you injury free, and to properly warm up joint, muscles and tendons and signal that more work is coming. Post exercise static stretching is also helpful for speeding up recovery and decreasing intensity of DOMS (delayed onset muscle soreness), which typically occurs a day or two after training.

Eat Enough of the Right Foods

Have you ever noticed that typically, as you age your appetite, or the amount you can consume at one sitting is reduced?

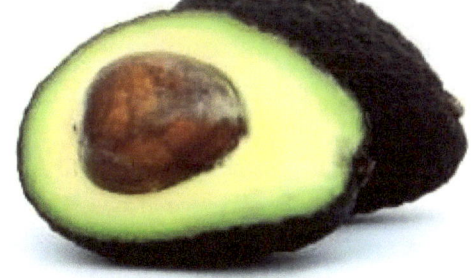

This is not necessarily a bad thing, but can become a problem in seniors when muscle atrophy accelerates and a mediocre diet becomes insufficient (actually leading to dietary deficiencies).

In such a scenario, there are two options:

Supplement With An Appetite Stimulant - these come in various types, be it prescription or over the counter, and work to improve appetite. Depending on your physical needs, you can take it either once or twice daily, to maximize your intake of calories through the day

Eat Calorie Heavy Foods - consume solid meals, loaded with protein and moderate amounts of good fat, and with low to moderate forms of slow digesting, fibrous carbs.

Doing so ensures that whatever is eaten is rich in nutritive value, and will be used for muscular synthesis and recovery. Consumption of a complete multi-vitamin/multi-mineral is also be advised to ensure micro nutritional deficiencies do not develop.

Fitness is the catalyst to the change initiated by a solid diet. You can compare following a diet plan without fitness to a car being supplied premium quality gas and lubricants, but not being serviced to improve/change its parts. The body is similar, as it needs to be maintained by partaking in regular exercise, which strengthens many structural components, and also promotes internal efficiency (AKA metabolism).

If you truly wish to live your life to the fullest, be sure to mold a lifestyle that incorporates solid fitness practices. You only have one life, make it count.

Other Health and Fitness Books by This Author

If you would like to read more about Health and Fitness, here is a list of the titles, CreateSpace links and descriptions:

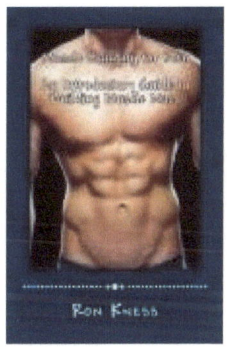

Muscle Building for Men – An Introductory Guide to Building Muscle Mass

https://www.createspace.com/5520238

In my book Muscle Building for Men – An Introductory Guide to Building Muscle Mass, I reveal a successful method of building muscle.

Your best bet is to formulate an all-over workout routine that helps you do three things:

• Burn fat
• Build muscle mass
• Strengthen your muscle

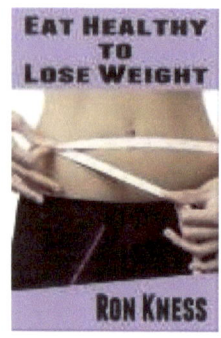

Eat Healthy to Lose Weight

https://www.createspace.com/4962939

As you read through our book, we show you which foods you should and should not be eating to reach your weight loss goal, along with discussing how to maintain your weight loss and stay within a few pounds of your goal weight. Banish the weight you keep gaining back each time by learning how to live a healthy lifestyle.

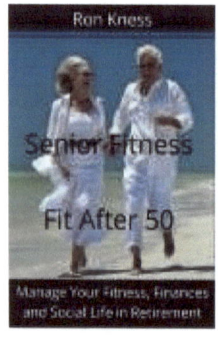

Senior Fitness – Fit After 50: Learn How to Manage Your Fitness, Finances and Social Life in Retirement

https://www.createspace.com/5474751

Inside you will discover answers to your most pressing questions:
• What do I need to know about downsizing my home?
• What are the best tips for staying healthy as you approach your 50's?
• When should I start planning for retirement?
• I am worried about being lonely once I retire, do others feel the same?
• Is it worthwhile to carry two homes during retirement?
And more…

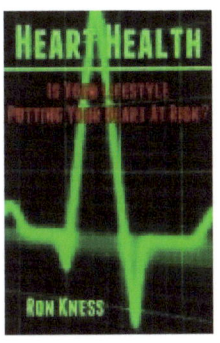

Heart Health: Is Your Lifestyle Putting Your Heart at Risk?

https://www.createspace.com/5464020

In my ebook Is Your Lifestyle Putting Your Heart At Risk? we discuss the six greatest risks to your heart and the lifestyle changes you can make to mitigate them.

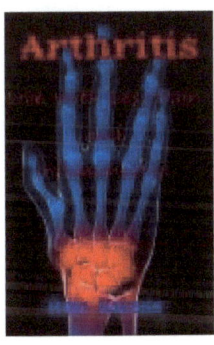

Arthritis – Live Wth Less Pain and Inflammation: Tips and Techniques You Can Use to Lessen the Pain and Inflammation

https://www.createspace.com/5457441

Discover Simple Tips & Information That Will Help Reduce The Painful Symptoms Of Arthritis!

You learn things like:
• Simple and effective information that will help you manage the pain and inflammation that comes along with arthritis, so that you can live an active, full life without debilitating pain.
• The different types of arthritis, their symptoms and how to alleviate their painful side effects.
• The pros and cons of over-the-counter arthritis medications, plus simple tips that will help you know how to choose the right supplements.

• Free, yet effective ways to get relief from arthritis pain and inflammation, so you don't have to suffer anymore.
the effects arthritis can have significant impact on your physical and mental well-being, but this books shows you how to overcome its painful symptoms and live life relatively pain free.

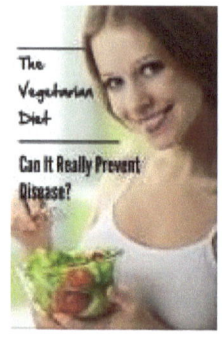

The Vegetarian Diet – Can It Really Prevent Disease?

https://www.createspace.com/5519874

Is a vegetarian diet right for you? Multiple studies have shown over and over that a vegetarian diet goes along way in preventing certain chronic diseases, such as:

• Heart Disease
• Cancer
• Diverticulitis
• Type 2 Diabetes
• Hypertension
• Obesity
• Kidney Failure

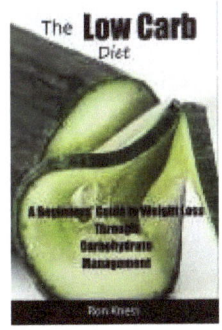

[The Low Carb Diet: A Beginner's Guide to Weight Loss Through Carbohydrate Management](#)

https://www.createspace.com/5416348

In my book "The Low-Carb Diet – A Beginners' Guide to Weight Loss Through Carbohydrate Management", I reveal a successful method of losing weight based in part on the amount and type of carbohydrates you consume.

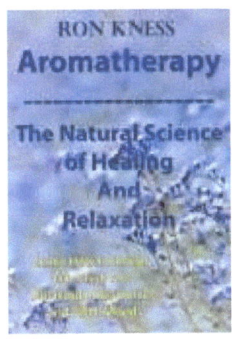

[Aromatherapy - The Science of Healing and Relaxation: Learn How Essential Oils Elicit The Relaxation Response And Alter Mood](#)

https://www.createspace.com/5714434

In my book Aromatherapy – The Science of Healing and Relaxation, we reveal the natural holistics methods you can use to heal the body from certain medical issues and to relive stress through relaxation. In particular we talk about:
• Aromatherapy - what it is and how it works
• Essential Oils – how the effects of certain aromas differs from others
• Recipes – how to make your own essential oil combinations

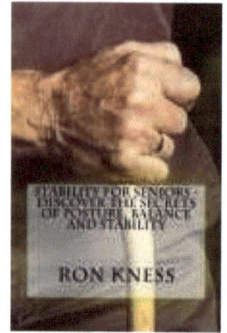

Stability for Seniors: Discover the Secrets of Posture, Balance and Stability

https://www.createspace.com/6096479

Many people sacrifice their health in pursuit of their career. They are so busy making a living that they neglect to make a life. The excuse that they do not have time to exercise is tossed about so frequently that they end up letting their health and fitness slide.

If you are not regularly active, you will have muscular atrophy over time. Your flexibility will decrease. Your core strength will diminish. As time progresses, you will be less limber and more rigid.

This is exactly how people age poorly. It's a process that has snowballed over time.

Only with regular exercise and a healthy diet can you have a body that is fit and has the ability to almost reverse aging.

If you have neglected your health for years and life seems to be a chore now because you can't get around without assistance, do not feel dejected.

You can remedy the situation. You can restore the strength, balance and stamina that you have lost. It is never too late to become what you might have been.

This guide will show you exactly what you need to do to restore your balance, strengthen your core and give you the ability to live life to its fullest. Read how …

About the Author

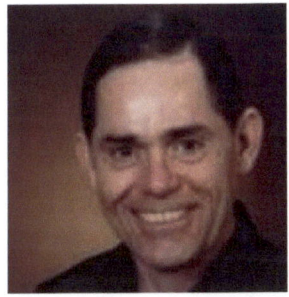

I grew up in Central Minnesota, where my parents owned and operated a fishing resort. Once out of high school I tried a couple of semesters of college, only to quit halfway through the Spring term; I decided at that time that college wasn't for me.

Then I decided to follow my father's previous occupation as an auto mechanic. I graduated from a two-year of vocational training course and worked as a mechanic for five years. While in vocational training, I decided to join the National Guard where I eventually ended up working full-time for 32 years.

So how does all of this relate to writing? In one of my leadership schools, the instructor, who was an English teacher at a juvenile detention center, presented writing to me in a whole new way - a way that started to develop my interest in working with words.

I eventually went back to college on the GI Bill while I was working and earned my Bachelor's degree in Business Administration. Taking a class or two per semester at night and on weekends took me seven years to complete my degree.

Fast forward about 40 years and I now have published over 75 books on Amazon for Kindle, CreateSpace and other publishing platforms.

Besides my own writing, I also ghostwrite ebooks, reports, articles, blogs and do Kindle conversions for clients on a variety of topics.

Today my wife and I are retired from our careers and live in Gold Canyon, AZ. I now write as a retirement business where you'll find me happily sitting in my office typing away on my laptop as I work on my next book or ghostwriting project . . . that is if we are not traveling on a cruise ship - our new-found mode of travel.

www.ingramcontent.com/pod-product-compliance
Lightning Source LLC
Chambersburg PA
CBHW040313010626
45792CB00022B/285